DO790273

Disclaimer

Medicine and nursing are continuously changing practices. The author and publisher have reviewed all information in this book with resources believed to be reliable and accurate and have made every effort to provide information that is up to date with best practices at the time of publication. Despite our best efforts we cannot disregard the possibility of human error and continual changes in best practices the author, publisher, and any other party involved in the production of this work can warrant that the information contained herein is complete or fully accurate. The author, publisher, and all other parties involved in this work disclaim all responsibility from any errors contained within this work and from the results from the use of this information. Readers are encouraged to check all information in this book with institutional guidelines, other sources, and up to date information. For up to date disclaimer information please visit: http://www.nrsng.com/about.

Photo Credits:
All photos are original photos taken or created by the author or rights purchased at Fotolia.com. All rights to appear in this book have been secured.

Some images within this book are either royalty-free images, used under license from their respective copyright holders, or images that are in the public domain. Images used under a creative commons license are duly attributed, and include a link to the relevant license, as per the author's instructions. All Creative Commons images used under the following license. All works in the public domain are considered public domain given life of the author plus 70 years or more as required by United States law.

The New Nurse Survival Guide

50 Tips to Survive and Thrive as a New Nurse

NRSNG.com | NursingStudentBooks.com

Jon Haws RN CCRN

Sandra Haws RD CNSC

TazKai LLC

Contents

Your Free Gift!

As a way of saying thanks for your purchase, I'm offering a free PDF download:

"63 Must Know NCLEX® Labs"

With these charts you will be able to take the 63 most important labs with you anywhere you go!

You can download the 4 page PDF document by clicking here, or going to NRSNG.com/labs

Introduction

Are you a brand new nurse? Are you just about to finish nursing school and preparing for the NCLEX®? Are you intimidated and just slightly overwhelmed by the stress of starting a new job and learning the culture of nursing?

You aren't alone.

The good news is there are tips and tricks that can help you excel in your career as a nurse. Many of those tips are so easy that it blows my mind new nurses aren't doing them.

In this book I will teach you 50 tips and tricks that you should implement as a new nurse to survive and thrive in your career.

You will find that by simply reviewing these tips and keeping them in mind you will find your first nursing job much more bearable. Will it still be hard? Of course. But with these tips you will have the knowledge, foresight, and skills you need to climb the mountain that is being a new nurse.

Think of me as your preceptor . . . I'm there to insure your success. We need more motivated, happy, hard working nurses, and I want you to succeed.

Who Am I?

My name is Jon Haws RN CCRN. I run the blog NRSNG.com, the NRSNG podcast, and I'm the author of dozens of books that help nurses and nursing students excel and raise above the pack. Once you have the tools nursing becomes so much easier.

Sick of spending hours and hours trying to find all the information you need for clinical and NCLEX® study? So was I . .

. . That's why I created NRSNG.com, a community of nurses and nursing students wanting to jump start their careers.

Come visit us at NRSNG.com or check in on Facebook.com/NRSNG.

Happy Nursing!

-Jon Haws RN CCRN

Explain Everything You Are Doing

Nurses dispense comfort, compassion, and caring without even a prescription.

-Val Saintsbury

Have you ever felt completely over your head? Imagine the last time you felt like you had no idea what was going on or what another person was talking about (first day of nursing school).I feel like this every time I talk to my father-in-law. He is an Aerospace Engineer, yep, an actual rocket scientist. I used to think I knew how batteries worked. Then I spoke with him. After a one hour conversation about batteries and how they work I realized I had no clue what he was talking about.

In a study by the US Department of Health and Human Services it was found that "Only 12 percent of U.S. adults had proficient health literacy" and "over a third of U.S. adults—77 million people—would have difficulty with common health tasks, such as following directions on a prescription drug label . . .".

As confused as I was about batteries, or how you may have felt the first day of nursing school, image how confused and frustrated our patients and their families must feel when physicians and nurses fail to properly explain what is going on or provide an explanation prior to drawing blood or hauling the patient of for a CAT scan (http://www.health.gov/communication/literacy/issuebrief/).

If you have spent any time in a hospital you know that nurses spend far more time with patients than any other health care professional. This means that the brunt of filling the gap between health literacy and explaining what is going on with the patient lies squarely on our shoulders. After the doctor zooms in and out of the room we are left to translate what was just said within our scope of practice.

I recently took care of a patient who had a pontine hemorrhage, a condition that presents with a mortality rate of 30-90% in otherwise healthy individuals, however, my patient had recently been diagnosed with liver disease making it nearly impossible for his blood to clot. Any attempt at saving this man's life was all but futile and the decision was made to manage his condition conservatively medically.

Vitamin K was ordered to aid in slowing the bleeding due to his inability to clot. When I told the family that I was giving him a shot to help him clot his blood a family member in the room with a self described "medical background" said, "Oh, are you giving him Heparin" . . . !

The point is, most of our patients and family members have no clue what is going on and for many of them the time they spend in the hospital will be one of the most scary, trying, horrifying events of their life. Rather than just sticking them to get blood, hauling them off to CAT scan, hanging a bag of antibiotics . . . take 30 seconds to explain in detail what you are doing and why.

This serves two purposes. It forces you to actually know what you are doing and why, which makes you a better nurse, and it eases tension and fears your patients and family might be feeling.

Be Honest With Managers

The character of a nurse is just as important as the knowledge he/she possesses.

-Carolyn Jarvis

Prior to becoming a nurse I worked in several other industries. Right before going to nursing school I worked as a buyer for a large sporting goods chain . . . "dream job" right? Not so much!

What I found in the business world was that it was very hard to speak openly with mangers about job satisfaction and career plans. Most co-workers were consigned to the fact that they would be in their current job until they died or their manager retired. There were so few opportunities that everyone was scared to take a risk and no one talked about it.

That isn't the case with nursing. With so many career paths, opportunities, and options it is well understood that the majority of nurses will be seeking new paths at some point in their career from grad school to education you can do almost anything with your career.

Because of this mobility it is possible speak very openly about plans with other nurses and managers. If you are struggling with your current schedule, role, or duties you should speak with your manager openly. If you are working hard and doing your best on the floor during your shifts your manager will trust your opinions and listen to your concerns.

After about a year on my floor and many bonus shifts and overtime I started to feel a bit exhausted. I spoke with my manager about my concerns and was able to work out a new schedule that works better for my family and my sanity.

A quick caveat . . . sadly there are still a handful of mistrusting managers out there. Prior to being too open it is important to make sure you know your manger and their personality.

Write PRN Meds Down

Some people think that doctors and nurses can put scrambled eggs back in the shell.

-Cass Canfield

It never fails . . . you are halfway through your shift everything is going great then suddenly your patient is in excruciating pain and needs treatment right away . . . there is no time to turn on your computer, wait for it to load, scroll through your patients medical record to find what pain medication is available and the schedule . . . they need relief now!

I learned very quickly in my career that I could save myself time and my patients moments of pain, nausea, anxiety, etc, by simply writing down all of the patients PRN medications as well as their dosing schedule and last administration at the very beginning of my shift prior to even seeing my patients.

Not only does this help in the above listed events, but it provides me with a chance to think through their plan of care and prepare myself to answer the inevitable question, "when can I have my pain meds?".

Below is the format of my "BRAIN" or the sheet I use to take report on my patient:

- Patient Information (name, allergies, code status, background, doctors)
- Body Systems Assessment
- Tasks to be Completed During my Shift (blood sugars, labs, tests)
- Meds
- PRN Meds (with next dose time)

Visit: NRSNG.com/54 for a free organization tool "BRAIN SHEET"

All of this information can be written down prior to even seeing the patient and puts you ahead of the game.

You Can't Control Patients or Their Outcomes

Our job as nurses is to cushion the sorrow and celebrate the job, everyday, while we are "just doing our jobs".

-Christine Belle

As a student nurse and a new nurse in a Neuro ICU I was always so worried about when I would have "my first medication error", or my first fall, or first code.

Unfortunately, I would stress over events that hadn't even occurred because I was so afraid of the potential outcome if/when it did occur. Beyond just insuring that alarms were set, medications were double checked, and critical patients were monitored very closely, I had a false sense of control and, for the lack of a better word, godly omnipotence over the events that would occur throughout my shift.

One night I was assigned to care for a patient who had already had three falls in another facility, and one in my facility. The patient was erratic and poorly oriented. As always, I made sure to set the bed alarm, I sat within viewing distance of his bed, and his wife agreed to spend the night and slept right next to his bed.

Halfway through the night, despite my best efforts and vigilance the patient found his way out of the bed. I felt terrible, I was crushed, how could one of MY patients fall.

A close friend on the floor could see that I was eating myself up about the incident and shared advice that has helped me cope with not only this event, but other unfortunate outcomes during my career.

flushes and alteplase flushes will be ordered to reestablish patent lines. Be sure to read the instructions thoroughly prior to administration of these medications and to follow hospital policy.

Upon completion of medication infusions flush all lines to maintain patency. This small tip will save you hours of headache during you career and insure you patient is able to receive the medication they need.

Flush Feeding Tubes

Apprehension, uncertainty, waiting, expectation, fear of surprise, do a patient more harm than any exertion.

-Florence Nightingale

O kay . . . so I have very few pet peeves as a nurse, but not flushing feeding tubes is one of them. Think for a minute about what we are infusing through these tubes (protein, carbs, fats), these are all things that can harden and clog very quickly and easily.

It seems to happen very often that we have chronically ill patients come in from other facilities for PEG tube revisions because the tubes were not properly flushed and now must be redone.

Flushing your PEGs, OG, and NG tubes is very easy to do and it is a good way to make sure all the food is flushed out of the line, that you have a patent line, and to give the patient a bit of fluids at the same time.

Check with your institution, many facilities have policies in place for how often and with how much fluid you should be flushing your feeding tubes. Some patients will also have orders to flush with a couple hundred of water Q6H or so.

Imagine for a moment that your ability to eat and receive nourishment were taken away from you. . . it would be terrible.

Eat and Pee

Nursing would be a dream job if there were no doctors.

-Gerhard Kocher

I have never understood nurses who say they don't have time to eat and pee during their shift. How long are you taking to pee?

The ICU that I work in is a busy downtown Trauma I hospital and I still find the time during each shift to take care of myself. That doesn't mean that I am taking a half hour lunch in the break room each shift, but I do grab a snack and a water bottle at a minimum if time is tight.

As far as going to the bathroom . . . seriously . . . how long DOES it take you to pee? A 12 hour shift equates to 720 minutes or 43,200 seconds. According to a recent study by Georgia Tech every mammal on earth takes an average of 21 seconds to pee (thanks Google). You can see the study here: http://www.huffingtonpost.com/2013/10/18/mammals-pee-21-seconds_n_4122906.html.

In my mind if you can't find time to relieve yourself during a shift you need to work on time management more than anything else.

With concern to eating. The best thing you can do is bring nutrient rich foods with you to work. Generally a Fiber One bar and a Naked or Bolthouse smoothie can fill you up real quick in just a matter of minutes.

You have to take care of yourself first to prevent burn out and insure you have the energy needed to complete the shift and come back for the next one.

Put Your Phone Away

Nurses may not be angels, but they are the next best thing!

-Unknown

I t seems strange that this is even something that needs to be mentioned, but nowadays our phones have almost become an extension of self that we can't go more than 2 seconds without looking at.

As a preceptor of students and new graduates I can tell you that nothing is more annoying than seeing a preceptee staring at their phone when there is work to do and mountains of information to learn.   Your social life can wait for a few hours.

I'm not suggesting that you don't bring your phone with you at all to work or that you never glance at it, but that you treat the job as a professional and make patient care and learning the number one priority. How much attention you give to your patients, their condition, and the learning process will show other nurses that you are engaged and willing to learn. Not only that but your capacity for learning is greatly increased when you give your full attention to learning.

Forbes.com states it this way:

"When you're trying to accomplish two dissimilar tasks, each one requiring some level of consideration and attention, multitasking falls apart. Your brain just can't take in and process two simultaneous, separate streams of information and encode them fully into short-term memory.

When information doesn't make it into short-term memory, it can't be transferred into long-term memory for recall later".

http://www.forbes.com/sites/douglasmerrill/2012/08/17/why-multitasking-doesnt-work/

Avoid Gossip Like the Plague

When you're a nurse you know that every day you will touch a life or a life will touch yours.

-Unknown

Do yourself a favor early on in your career and make a vow that you will never get involved in the gossip, back biting, or secrets that will spread around your floor.

With time it seems that hospital floors become a quasi family with each nurse playing a different role. With this it is practically inevitable that gossip will start to arise. Not only that, but floors will begin to gossip about other floors. There seems to be a rivalry in my hospital between the different ICUs and between nurses on almost every floor.

You will go much further in your career and be much happier at work if you just assume that every nurse is working their hardest and doing their best to take care of patients. Simply assume that no nurse is out there just to make your job harder.

Worrying about yourself and letting the actions of other nurses just roll of your back will help tremendously in your career.

Develop Thick Skin

Save one life and you're a hero, save one hundred lives and you're a nurse.

-Unknown

As a new nurse you are going to be under a lot of pressure from patients, families, managers, preceptors, doctors, other medical staff, and yourself. It will be impossible to live up to the expectations of each of these individuals at the same time and trying to do so will result in you falling apart.

It is sad, but there are still many nurses and doctors that are unable to have a civilized conversation with other human beings. Patients and their family members are going through one of the most difficult challenges of their lives. Other nurses are just as stressed as you. All this compounds to result in some pretty heavy conversations.

There are usually three outcomes I've seen when you combine these settings. The new nurse learns to just brush it all off and keep about their business, the new nurse internalizes all the negativity and breaks, and lastly the new nurse begins to fight back and becomes part of the problem.

It is always sad to me when I see new, young nurses encounter their first real stressful situation with a patient and a doctor yelling conflicting orders at them. I always pray a little that they will become strong and learn to roll with the punches.

When I began my internship there was another young nurse in my group. This was her first job. She was excited and looking forward to changing the world. Shortly into our internship I could see that the pressure and negativity that can abound in health care was starting to break her down. After many shifts that ended up with her crying in the staff bathroom I could see her begin to change. Within a couple months the yelling, the negativity, and the sheer difficulty of being a nurse no longer seemed to break her down.

It's okay to cry, it's okay to feel overwhelmed, it's okay to feel exhausted and not want to come back, but to succeed and raise above all the negativity and difficulty of the job you will need to develop thick skin and let all the negativity roll off of you.

Memorize and Write Down Important Phone Numbers

Keep your thoughts positive because your thoughts become your words. Keep your words positive because your words become your behavior. Keep you behavior positive because your behavior becomes your habits. Keep you habits positive because your habits become your values. Keep your values positive because your values become your destiny.

-Mahatma Gandhi

Having a collection of the right phone numbers will save your life as a nurse.

To do your job well you will need to rely on so many other individuals (doctors, xray, respiratory, secretary, charge nurse, pharmacy, lab, admitting, pt, and so many more).

I HATE talking on the phone . . . in fact, I never turn the volume up on my phone when I'm not at work. My wife, family, and friends know that if they want to reach me they are going to have to send a text. As a nurse I have had to learn to appreciate and embrace talking on the phone because being a patient advocate requires organizing care between so many other individuals that on some shifts the majority of your time is spent talking on the phone.

With this in mind let me tell you that you need to have a card that is attached to your name badge that has the most important phone numbers on it and you need to keep your hospital phone on you and turned on at all times during your shift.

I work on an enormous ICU where at times nurses can be isolated in far corners of the floor. If things take a turn for the worst and you do not know the phone numbers of those you need to reach you will be out of luck. Be a patient advocate and keep your phone on you at all times and have the numbers you need to know written down or memorized.

Identify Your Patients #1 Risk

People will forget what you said, they will forget what you did, but they will never forget how you made them feel!

-Maya Angelou

One thing I do with all new nurses and nursing students before we even enter the patients room the first time is make them identify the patients biggest risk.

What do we need to be focusing on during this shift to keep our patient safe?

Is it hemodynamics, neuro status, safety? What are they at most risk for and what do we need to make our priority when monitoring this patient.

As nurses we cannot control or predict what will happen during the 12 hours we are with the patient, but we can make educated guesses and set precautions based on trends and our knowledge of the patients and their disease processes in attempt to keep them safe and avoid unnecessary turns for the worst.

If you are taking care of a patient with severe COPD exacerbation who refuses to keep the bi-PAP on and is becoming increasingly lethargic you need to obviously focus on their respiratory status. Making a defined mental note, setting alarms, letting other nurses know, notifying RT, and sitting close to the patient are all simple things you can do to focus on their #1 risk factor. This helps you to cut through the clutter and focus on what is MOST important (sound like nursing school again?).

In the ideal world we would be able to focus on all of our patients needs at the same time however, being a wise nurse you are able to focus on the ABCs first and then prioritize other care once your patient is safe. You will find you are more organized, less stressed, and more able to provide holistic care to your patients as you approach your care this way.

Keep in mind that a patients #1 risk factor might change multiple times during a shift . . . hence the nursing assessment.

Show Up Ready for the Hardest Shift - Every Shift!

It is not how much you do, but how much love you put in the doing.

-Mother Theresa

You will have shifts as a nurse that will push you to your breaking point. As you walk out after the shift you will honestly question why you ever decided to be a nurse and consider never coming back.

This is the reality of being a nurse. We work in a tremendously UNpredictable field. So much of what we do is so far out of our control that it is almost impossible to plan or anticipate.

Since we cannot control this, I find it best to anticipate that each time you walk into the hospital doors you might be showing up to the hardest shift of your life . . . anything less than that is bonus!

I do not feel that looking at it this way is pessimistic, but simply a way to prepare your mind for what might lay ahead of you. Just remind yourself that a shift is only 12 hours, you are strong enough that you can do anything for 12 hours.

One thing that has really helped me with this is a simple ritual. As I pull of the highway on my drive to work I roll my car window down and put on a song that I listen to before each shift this helps me get my mind in the right place and prepare myself for the shift ahead.

Find a ritual that you can do prior to each shift to get your mind in the right place and prepare yourself for anything that might be thrown at you during the next 12 hours.

Leave Home at Home

To know even one life has breathed easier because you have lived, that is to have succeeded.

-Ralph Waldo Emerson

Shortly after getting married my wife and I took a job at the same company. For the most part this was an awesome deal. We worked the same schedule, car pooled, get to spend a lot of time together. But, whenever we had a disagreement at home it was really hard to just forget about it when I was at work.

Nursing can be a very stressful job that requires us to give a lot of ourselves when we are at work. Nurses are human so we are all dealing with stress of our own. To be able to give of ourselves, provide care to our patients, and make it through a tough shift it is important to leave personal stress at home.

Here are a few things I have done to help with this:

Don't live close to work - on my days off I am not having to drive past work and think about the stresses. During my drive to work I have the chance to leave home at home and begin to focus on the shift and what needs to be done while at work.

Work back to back shifts - this isn't possible for some, but I find that working all my shifts back to back allows me to have "my work days and my home days". My family and friends know that when I am in work mode I am mostly unreachable. This also gives me 4-5 days at home to deal with the stresses of home without the interruption of work.

Keep my work stuff at work - I keep my name badge, stethoscope, and other "work" things at work. This way when I show up for a shift and begin to put those things on I am slipping into work mode and leaving other stresses behind.

Take a minute to get my mind right - if I am having a particularly hard time leaving a problem at home I will sit in the parking lot for just a moment once I get to work and listen to a favorite song as I think about the shift. This provides a slow transition into work mode and helps me focus on what I need to be thinking about to take care of my patients.

Check IV Drug Compatibility

To do what nobody else will do, in a way that nobody else can do, in spite of all we go through: that is what it means to be a nurse.

-Rawsi Williams

I know, this might seem like an obvious one, but in the heat of the moment when you are hanging multiple pressors, bicarb, antibiotics, and keppra you might not be thinking about compatibility and worrying more about getting the medications into your patient.

Some medications don't mix well and can crystallize or worse when run through the same IV. This isn't always a concern, but if you only have one IV site, or if you are trying to hang 6 or more drugs at the same time (it happens), then you will start to run into compatibility issues.

You facility should have a resource available for you to check IV drug compatibilities. When I am caring for very sick patients and I know I will be hanging multiple medications I usually just bring the resource up on my computer at the beginning of my shift.

I am most familiar with the King Guide, but you should find out what your facility uses and become a super user. If you take over a patient with multiple medications running through one IV take a minute and check compatibility. This isn't to catch the off going nurse in error but to keep you and your patient safe. Once you take over the patient it is your license on the line.

Arrive on Time

A nurse will always give us hope, an angel with a stethoscope.

-Terri Guillemets

Not a lot to say here. Just arrive on time or early for your shift. This helps you in a few ways:

- Gives you time to get your mind right
- Gives you time to get a good report
- Shows other nurses respect
- That's just what adults do when they have a job

It just blows my mind when nurses show up at the last possible moment for a shift or continually show up late. When you are a new nurse your goal should be to arrive to your shift before your preceptor. This shows them that you are taking your job seriously and eager to learn.

According to a study from Penn State University, arriving late to work is a sign of withdrawal behaviors demonstrating that an employee is unhappy with their job. This message is conveyed to managers, charge nurses, and preceptors. What message are you conveying?

https://wikispaces.psu.edu/display/PSYCH484/13.+Withdrawal+Behaviors

Humility and Confidence vs Hubris

The way we communicate with others and with ourselves
ultimately determines the quality of our lives.

-Anthony Robbins

There is nothing more encouraging than a confident yet humble new grad. There is nothing more discouraging than a new nurse full of hubris. What's hubris?

Hubris is defined as excessive pride or self-confidence.

Self-confidence is good. **Excessive** pride or self-confidence is terrifying in a new nurse.

I am always horrified when I see a brand new nurse not ask questions, state that they don't need help, or remain quiet during an entire shift. The scary thing behind this is that I remember what it was like being a new nurse. I had done extremely well in school and studied very hard yet there was so much that I didn't know and without the help of a patient preceptor I would have been completely lost.

When new nurses walk into a unit full of hubris I wish I could just ask them to leave.

To me a confident nurse is willing to try new things, speaks clearly when talking with doctors, is not afraid to admit what they don't know and recognizes their limitations and is quick to ask for help when needed.

I would take one confident and humble nurse over 5 nurses full of hubris any day and deal with the staffing issue myself. To work as a team and to learn and grow as an individual nurse and as a unit you need staff willing to learn, confident in their skills, and smart enough to recognize when they need help.

Be a Person to Your Patients

To accomplish great things, you must not only act, but also dream, not only plan, but also believe.

-Anatole France

It's funny to even write this tip, but I can tell you from experience that many nurses forget to simply be a person.

This doesn't mean being unprofessional but simply letting them know that you are a person too and not just a machine that has no feelings. Patients and family members want to know that you care about them and that you want the best for them. A simple way to do this is to just find a piece of common ground with your patient or their family.

You're primary focus is still patient care and educating them on their disease process but this can be done with finesse, showing them that you are a person and are genuinely interested in their well being.

Are you from the same area?

Do you both have dogs?

Do you both have kids?

Have you both traveled to the same place?

Is there a beautiful sunset you can talk about?

Do you like the same restaurant?

You need to be careful when talking with patients about yourself. There is a fine line between sharing about yourself and displaying yourself as unprofessional and uncaring.

If you share too much or monopolize conversation patients may see you as unknowledgeable or just plain rude.

You should also avoid sharing strong opinions (politics, religion, etc). In an article on MedScape they state:

"Sharing strong beliefs or emotions without understanding the patient's perspective seems risky; a practitioner may unknowingly infuse the dialogue with his or her needs without carefully tying them to the patient's needs..."
http://www.medscape.com/viewarticle/568390

When it comes down to it, the most important component is that the patient and family feel that you care about them. Learning to ask the right questions and share the right information comes with time but don't be afraid to share a little about yourself.

Take Days Off

I'm not telling you it's going to be easy, I'm telling you it's going to be worth it.

-Art Williams

Sounds easy right? Well for some reason you run into nurses that have hundreds and hundreds of PTO hours banked and just refuse to take any time off.

I personally don't understand it. During my first six months or so on the job I didn't take any time off and actually worked extra shifts because I wanted to learn everything that I could while I was still brand new. I am a firm believer in accelerated learning by complete immersion.

After those first six months or so I took time off to just simply be at home more with my family or to go camping and to take my mind off the hospital. Without this precious time off I would have completely burnt out.

If you work your schedule right you can actually have 8 days off without even using a vacation day. You can also get two weeks off by only using 3 vacation days. To do this just work the first three days of the first week and the last three of the next week.

I would do this quiet a bit during my first year to provide me with time to relax and unwind. This helps you refresh and gives you the energy you need to hit the ground running when you return to work. I think a lot of young nurses burn out because they don't take the needed time off to just relax and rejuvenate. You don't even need to go anywhere fancy (this usually adds stress anyway). Just spend more time at home with the family or outside.

Look Doctors in the Eyes

I am only one, but still I am one. I cannot do everything, but still I can do something, and because I cannot do everything I will not refuse to do something that I can do.

-Helen Keller

When a doctor assumes the care of a patient they take a personal investment in the outcome of the patients care just like we do as nurses. When the doctor leaves at night or steps away to see another patient they assume that you as a nurse has the knowledge and skills to take care of the nurse as a professional.

To instill confidence in the physician and to participate as part of an interdisciplinary team look the doctor in the eyes. Not only that, but you need to speak up and defend your decisions. As nurses we come from a different education base than physicians but we have the same goal, the patients outcome. We sit at the patients bedside and have a unique perspective on what is occurring with the patient.

Eye contact shows general respect, instills confidence, and helps you to take confidence in your work and your skills.

Hospitals are Small

The trained nurse has become one of the great blessings of humanity, taking a place beside the physician and the priest....

-William Osler

Thought you would get away from gossip, reputations, and popularity contests when you left high school? Think again.

I work at a large Level I Trauma center in a large metropolitan area and I can tell you that hospitals are very small places and people get to know each other and reputations spread.

How do you want to be known?

Between units, specialties, management, and throughout the hospital people will start to get to know you and your reputation will go wherever you go.

I am certainly not a proponent of brownnosing and sucking up, but I do believe strongly in working your hardest and doing a good job in all that you do. When you go to work you are leaving your name on everything you do. Don't dirty your name. You never know when you will want to change jobs, change floors, or need a recommendation from a manager. Just do your best every time you go to work and be friendly and learn all that you can.

Get Some Sleep

Bound by paperwork, short on hands, sleep, and energy... nurses are rarely short on caring.

-Sharon Hudacek

Prior to my first night shift I was terrified I would fall asleep halfway through. I remember packing loads of caffeine and snacks to try to keep myself awake. Luckily I didn't fall asleep and I have found a few tricks to help with the awkward sleep cycle.

Working three shifts in a row works best for me as a night nurse. This allows me to basically divide my week into two sections; human mode and zombie mode.

When I am off work I am able to adjust quickly to a "normal" sleep schedule and spend time with my family.

When I am in zombie mode my family and friends know not to call or disturb me during the day because I will be curled up in my bed getting what sleep I can.

Prior to working a three day stent I have found the best thing to do the day prior to going to work is to stay up a bit late or wake up extra early, I usually wake up at like 4:30am and go for a jog the day I work my first night shift.

I then go to sleep at around 11am and sleep until about 5pm. This gives me 5-6 hours of sleep before my shift and allows me enough time to eat a normal meal and get ready without rushing.

When I get home from work after a night shift I'll usually be in bed by 9 or 10am and try to sleep until 5pm. Some days I have more luck than others sleeping between shifts.

If I really just can't sleep I'll watch a movie in bed, read, or take a bath or something relaxing that at least allows my body to rest.

After my last shift on a three day stent I come home and head straight to bed and sleep until noon or 1pm. I then awake from the dead and try to have as normal an afternoon as possible. Waking at noon allows me to get to bed at a normal time on my first day off.

This is the sleep schedule that works for me. Find what works for you and experiment a bit until you find something that works well. Whatever you do be sure to get enough sleep to function both at work and at home. I have been able to do the night shift with a family and other responsibilities. You can make it work too.

Even if you aren't working the night shift, get enough sleep. Adequate sleep will help you better manage the stress of nursing and help you to learn quicker and easier.

Know Your Patients Vital Sign Trends at Any Moment

Panic plays no part in the training of a nurse.

-Elizabeth Kenny

W hat were the patients vital signs over night? You better be able to answer that question from the top of your head without needing to run to the computer or find a flow sheet.

I personally feel that if you can't tell me what your patients VS are at any given moment, you aren't taking care of your patient.

In the ICU patients are hemodynamically unstable. At a minimum we are monitoring BP every 15 minutes and documenting vitals every hour. Many patients are on vasoactive drips and suffering from disease processes that greatly affect their hemodynamic stability. If a nurse is unable to, at any moment, state their patients vital signs, what are they doing taking care of that patient? Can you tell I'm a bit serious about this?

Mentally taking note every couple minutes of your patients vital signs will come with time but make it a priority from the start.

When you are trying to learn how to chart, manage time, and start an IV, it can become easy to lose track of what really matters . . . the patients well being. Our most reliable source for determining the patients well being is the nursing assessment, vital signs, and labs.

Seasoned nurses have learned how to monitor vital signs and keep them stored in the back of their minds at all times.

If you don't work in an ICU or if you have aids taking your vital signs you had BETTER be reviewing what they find. It is your job as the nurse to interpret the data the techs record. They may not report vitals that are outside the normal range. If you give lisinopril without first looking at the blood pressure you are not providing safe care.

Look at, review, and know your patients vital signs!

Don't Trust SpO$_2$

You know you're a nurse if... you triage the laundry when at home: This pile needs immediate attention, the pile can wait, this pile, with a little stain stick will be OK until you get back to it.

-Donna Wilk Cardillo

What is SpO$_2$? Can you tell me what it is measuring?

SpO$_2$ is basically a measure of the percentage of hemoglobin binding sites occupied by oxygen. Unfortunately, this doesn't necessarily tell us about end organ oxygenation. SpO2 is helpful as a general indicator of oxygenation but if you begin to rely on this number over your nursing assessment you have made a mistake.

Patients can compensate and machines can fail. If your assessment and nursing judgment tell you that your patient is struggling to breath it is time to take more invasive measurements to determine true respiratory status.

Oxygen is transported in two ways; bound to hemoglobin (SpO2 [peripherally]/SaO2 [arterially]) and dissolved in the plasma (PaO2). SpO2 is an indirect measure while the SaO2 obtained via an ABG is a direct measure. Falsely relying on an indirect measure like SpO2 can highly alter quick intervention in poorly oxygenated patients.

More appropriate numbers for judging respiratory status are:

SvO2: mixed venous O2, how much circulating oxygen the tissues are extracting

SaO2: oxygen saturation of arterial blood

Obviously, this is a more complex and in depth discussion for an entirely different book, but the short lesson is . . . don't rely on the PulseOx more than your nursing assessment and judgment.

Look Up Labs

Nurses — one of the few blessings of being ill.

-Sara Moss-Wolfe

Labs can slip in to your patients records completely unnoticed. Unless a value is far out of normal range the lab usually won't call you. It thus becomes the duty of the nurse to look into the patients chart to review laboratory data.

I've seen patients remain on contact isolation for days because of "C-diff" even after the results come back negative because no one ever looked back at the chart to review the lab result.

Even if you don't understand the correlation between lab values and the patients condition it can be very helpful to you to review the data as this will help you in becoming familiar with normal values for your hospital as well as help you in beginning to make connections between disease processes and expected lab data.

So, at the beginning of each shift take a minute and look up the most recent lab data. If you run a stat lab during your shift be sure to review it. If you draw morning or scheduled labs on your patient be sure to go back into the chart and take a peek at the results about an hour or so after.

You should do this with CT scans, MRIs, and other diagnostic testing as well. Not only will this help in your learning but doctors and other nurses will ask about recent labs and it is nice to have the information available.

The Power of Yet

Nursing is not for everyone. It takes a very strong, intelligent, and compassionate person to take on the ills of the world with passion and purpose and work to maintain the health and well-being of the planet. No wonder we're exhausted at the end of the day!

-Donna Wilk Cardillo

Sadly, as humans we like to judge ourselves based on what we either are or aren't. We don't leave much room for growth and achievement when it comes to accepting ourselves and judging ourselves.

Learning to apply the word "yet" to our view of ourselves is a powerful way to find increased ability to grow and accept ourselves.

Listen to these two statements.

"I can't start IVs."

"I can't start IVs yet."

Each of these statements essentially says the same thing, but applying the word yet to the end of the second statement suggests that this individual sees themselves as a being in progress rather than a failure (like the first).

This concept of YET comes from psychologist Carol Dweck. When I heard her talk about this concept in a recent TED talk in resonated very strongly with me. You can view the video here: http://www.ted.com/talks/carol_dweck_the_power_of_believing_that_you_can_improve?language=en

When approaching a problem or thinking about who you are, think are you not smart enough to solve the problem or have you just not solved it YET?

Nursing is an ever changing field. You can learn the tricks, skills, and science required to be a great nurse, but understand that we are all evolving beings with so much to learn and achieve.

Simply applying this one little word in your life gives you the power to achieve extraordinary things.

Internship is the Time to Learn

Nurses are the hospitality of the hospital.

-Carrie Latet

If you are lucky enough to obtain your first job in a hospital that offers internships you will be given an extended time to learn and adjust to life as a nurse.

There is so much to learn when you start out as a nurse.

It is an entirely new culture. Learning how to chart, manage your time, set priorities, and basic nursing sciences can be extremely stressful to say the least.

Internships provide you with a preceptor and standardized learning to help you adjust to life as a new nurse.

While I was a new intern I spent the majority of my time off reading focused materials that dealt with the disease processes I was seeing on my floor.

Take advantage of this time to learn everything that you can while you have a focused teacher right next to you. Use every resource your hospital has to learn as much as you can.

If you are placed in a short term internship do what you can to absorb all that you can. As your time in internship begins to dwindle down if you are not feeling prepared to be on your own as a nurse take a minute and speak with your manager and preceptor and ask for additional time.

Don't Waste All Your Money

I may be compelled to face danger, but never fear it, and while our soldiers can stand and fight, I can stand and feed and nurse them.

-Clara Barton

It's always fun (sad) to watch new co-workers start their first job and begin to spend their money. I was recently talking with a co-worker who told me that her eating out/bar tab bill came to $750 per month. During the same conversation she told me that she was struggling to make her rent payment and that she had to adjust her student loan payments.

Point of the story is, when you start that first job you will feel like you are rolling in money. You will be so used to spending like a student and living on Ramen Noodles that initially the paychecks will start to pile up a bit in your bank account and slowly you will start to spend it. First on new scrubs, then new shoes, before you know it all that piled up money will be gone and you will be struggling to pay back your student loans.

In a 2012 study it was found that about 50% of Americans spend more than they earn (http://www.huffingtonpost.com/2012/05/17/americans-spending-more-than-they-earn_n_1523920.html). Spending less than you earn and saving your money can be very hard and it takes a lot of discipline but the rewards add up quickly as you stash more money away. Soon you will find that unlike your peers your loans are paid off, you have money saved, and you are no longer stressing over money.

A couple websites and podcasts that might help with money management are:

- Suze Orman Show
- Mr. Money Moustache
- Dough Roller Podcast

Pay Off Your Student Loans

How can anybody hate nurses? Nobody hates nurses. The only time you hate a nurse is when they're giving you an enema.

-Warren Beatty

When I graduated nursing school my student loan bill was just about $60,000. Yeah, I went to a private nursing program.

To say that this felt a bit overwhelming would be a major understatement. I felt like I was buried in a huge mountain of debt.

I was lucky enough to get a job right out of school. To help make extra money I worked the night shift and picked up as many weekend shifts as possible. After finishing internship I picked up all the overtime I was allowed. Within less than a year I had paid off over $40,000 of the debt.

When approaching debt I think it is best to focus on the highest interest loans first. The longer you hang on to high interest loans the more that loan is going to cost you.

My wife and I organized all of my loans from highest interest to lowest interest and just went to town paying them off. For a year we lived with my parents, we had two kids, it wasn't easy. Once we paid off every loan that was more than 4% interest we slowed down and started saving money.

If you have a hard time finding a job, most loans provide a six month grace period were you are not required to pay off the loan. However, keep in mind that even though you aren't making payments, interest is still accruing on those loans.

There are programs that offer income based repayment programs as well. Again, any time you decrease or stop your payment . . . you don't stop the interest from piling up.

If you have the money for vacations, expensive designer scrubs, a new car, furniture, or eating out, then you have the money to get rid of your loans.

Keep in mind that even small adjustments in interest rates make enormous differences in the lifetime cost of your loan. Extending the term, cutting the cost, combining loans will all end up costing you.

Try this website to figure out what a loan will actually cost you: http://www.bankrate.com/calculators/managing-debt/annual-percentage-rate-calculator.aspx

Verify Information Given in Report

It would not be possible to praises nurses too highly.

-Stephen Ambrose

The nursing handoff report is when the off going nurse communicates the essential information with the oncoming nurse. This is an important time for you to get the vital information, head to toe assessment, family dynamics, and physician orders from the nurse who just spent 12 hours with your patient.

Unfortunately, it can result in a game of "telephone" (remember the old game from childhood) as the patient spends more and more time in the hospital. What begins as an order to "keep SBP >120" can turn into "only feed the patient greenbeans on Wednesdays". This becomes more of a problem with complex patients and patients who have extended stays in the hospital.

Take a minute before each shift to skim through the orders and to verify them with what you were told in handoff report. When in doubt always go with what the written order states.

In a rush it is easy as a nurse to miss orders, forget orders, and just skip over important orders.

RT Should Be Your Best Friend

It's a beautiful thing when career and passion come together.

-Anonymous

N o one is going to have your back more than your respiratory therapist. RTs are trained in the management of vents and respiratory treatments. When your patient starts to decline chances are you will have an RT right at your side.

The first phone number you need to learn and have on your speed dial is the number for your RT. Get to know those that work your shift and be friendly to them. If your patient start to quickly desat or you just don't feel comfortable about their respiratory status you want to have an RT that knows you and is quick to the bedside to help.

How To Find Your First Job

Your work is going to fill a large part of your life, and the only way to be truly satisfied is to do what you believe is great work. And the only way to do great work is to love what you do. If you haven't found it yet, keep looking. Don't settle.

-Steve Jobs

One of the biggest questions nursing students ask is, "When should I start looking for a job?".

This can be a difficult question to answer and will vary depending on the job market you are in. I will share with you tips on finding that first job, but every job market will be different based on how many nursing schools there are, how many hospitals there are, if internships are offered, and so many other factors.

First of all, most hospitals won't show much interest in student nurses. Once you have RN after your name you will find that the responses to your search will increase greatly. It is possible to begin applying to jobs a month or two before graduation but I wouldn't send out applications before that.

Take the NCLEX as soon as you graduate and feel prepared. You don't need to be scoring 100% on practice exams to take the NCLEX. Remember a PASS is all you need.

Prior to beginning your search identify where you WANT to work. Do you want to work in an ED, ICU, NICU, or do you really not care?

Next identify if you want to work in a large hospital or a small community hospital.

Lastly, spend time working on and fine tuning your resume and interview skills. Send it to people you know and practice common interview questions out loud so that you are comfortable answering questions with confidence.

With all of this in mind you are now armed for your search.

Start with Google.

Begin by searching for "internship" "residency" "new nurse" "graduate nurse" "nurse resident" jobs in the area that you live. These are the most common words used to post jobs for new nurses.

Do the same search with Indeed.com.

Once you have identified those facilities that offer these types of positions work backwards to find an email or phone number for a nurse recruiter. You can also do a Google search for nurse recruiter _____ hospital. Your goal here is to obtain contact information for anyone that can answer basic questions for you about the best time to apply, how many applicants, what specific things they are looking for etc.

If you are unable to find this contact information see if the hospital has a special site or Facebook page for their internships. Some large hospitals in my area have a dedicated Facebook page just for their new nurse programs.

Apply to each of these programs in the area that you want to work. Then . . . here's the key apply to other jobs at other hospitals as well. As a new grad experience counts more than anything and waiting for that "perfect job" and the "perfect hospital" can do you a lot of harm as you are letting time pass by without experience. You GOAL is to get that one job that you want but in reality you are willing to take any job at this point.

Attend every job fair you can find. Go directly to hospitals and attempt to speak face to face with nurse recruiters to find out the best time to apply to internships.

Above ALL else . . . exhaust every connection that you have. If you know nurses that are already working in hospitals ask them for a reference, many times they will even get a referral bonus. Never underestimate the power of a good friend and a good reputation. Nurse managers are far more willing to hire the friend of a good working nurse than to take a chance on a random hire.

Most importantly don't get too down on yourself. Be relentless about finding that first job. My hospital receives about 800 applications for just 40 internship spots. A lot of it comes down to prescreening and just pure luck.

If time continues to pass without finding a job you can attempt to find a position in another city or state, you can get your ACLS or other certifications that do not require experience. Just don't give up and keep refining your process. With each position that you do not receive try to determine what it was that resulted in you not getting the job . . . then fix that for the next application.

Avoid Action Illusion

Nurses have come a long way in a few short decades. In the past our attention focused on physical, mental and emotional healing. Now we talk of healing your life, healing the environment, and healing the planet.

-Lynn Keegan

One of the ways that we can waste a lot of time both in nursing school and as a nurse is through the habit of action illusion. This term action illusion comes from the book 'Mind Gym', and what it basically means is that we can get into a habit of busying ourselves with activities that don't actually help get the job done.

In the instance of school for example we can bring all of our notes, bring all of our books, highlight a bunch of pages, take a bunch of notes, et cetera, and just busy ourselves doing a bunch of things that aren't actually helping us to learn the material.

In the instance of work, one thing that I often see a lot of nurses do is busy themselves with a tremendous amount of tasks that aren't actually helping them to take care the patient or get the job done. What can help best in avoiding action illusion is to take a minute and plan ahead what you're going to be doing. Now, it can be tricky because planning can also become part of action illusion, if we plan too long then we actually are just wasting time.

What you need to do is sit back, identify what the key tasks are that need to be done, and then find the quickest way to do those. There's no point in taking longer than what you need to take to get a task done. For example, starting in IV, and delaying it, and delaying it, and delaying it. If you need to start the IV figure out exactly what you need to get, exactly when you're going to do it, and then go and take care of the job.

Piddling around and wasting time with other unimportant tasks that aren't going to help you get that job done is action illusion. The reason action illusion happens is because it makes us feel like we're being busy, we feel our lives with things that help us to feel busy, when in reality we're just wasting time.

To help you with action illusion, I would suggest reading the book 'Mind Gym', this is a book that provides a bunch of different mental exercises and tools and tricks to help you better take control of your habits and your mind. Time management is one of the most important tasks that you can learn. Be cognizant and take a look and take the time to evaluate if you're just doing things to look busy and to make yourself think you're being busy, or if the actual tasks that you're doing are actually important to getting your job done.

Seek Opportunities

To do what nobody else will do, a way that nobody else can do,
in spite of all we go through; that is to be a nurse.

– Rawsi Williams, BSN, RN

One of the reasons I went into nursing in the first place was because there's so many opportunities with nursing, once you get that RN after your name you can become a teacher, you can work in law, you can work in business, you can work at the bed side, you can work in management, there's just so much that can be done as a nurse. With that in mind it's important to make sure that you're taking advantage of every opportunity that arises.

As a student nurse, when you're on your floor during clinicals make sure you're approaching other nurses and asking about different things that they have going on, ask if they have any procedures that need to be done. Ask if they have any different charting that you haven't experienced that needs to be done. Once you enter internship as a new nurse make sure that you continue to do this, if you get all the work done that you need to with your patients, walk around the unit and ask other nurses if they have any work that they need help with.

Seeking these opportunities and taking advantage of these opportunities, you begin to learn in a much faster rate. You're going to be exposed to much more, and you're going to see new things. The more times you start an IV, the more it's going to become second nature. The more times you're able to take care of a patient with the ventilator, the more it's going to become second nature.

Seek every opportunity you can to be exposed to new situations and to learn.

This knowledge is only going to help you be a standout with your peers, and it will help you to be better prepared to take care of your patients.

This will help advance your career, advance your knowledge, and advance your skill sets.

Arrive on Time

Panic plays no part in the training of a nurse.

— Sister Elizabeth Kenny

Arriving on time for your shift plays a couple different important roles. First of all, arriving on time allows you to get in the right mindset when you get to work. Sometimes when I arrive to work, I'll just sit in my car for a minute, listen to a song that gets me in the right mindset and prepares me to be able to take care of my patients and to just leave the stresses of home, and life aside, so that I can give myself at work.

Timely arrival allows you to research about your patients, to look at their vital sign trends, to read over some of their history, and some of the progress knows that the physicians have written so that when you walk into the room the first time it's not all brand new to you it gives you that time to learn about the patient and be prepared to take care the patient.

Arriving on time allows the nurse that you're getting report from to have time to give a good report and get out on time. It shows respect to your co-workers and what goes around comes around.

Figuring out what time to leave your home to get to work can take a little experimenting. I have figured out what time I need to leave down to a science depending on what day I am working.

Accept Feedback

The most important practical lesson than can be given to nurses is to teach them what to observe.

– Florence Nightingale

As I mentioned before I can be a prideful person, when I'm in a situation of being precepted or being mentored I always respect my preceptor, my mentor, but sometimes I can have a hard time accepting feedback.

I like to receive the feedback and it's very helpful to me to be able to learn and to grow when I but it can be hard for me to sit there and take that feedback when it's constructive and showing me where maybe I need to improve. That can be hard for most people.

However, getting this feedback from an experienced nurse can be very helpful in you understanding areas of opportunity that you can improve, and that you can grow upon. With your preceptor, with your mentor, with your manager, understand that these are nurses that are coming from more experience, they understand what it takes to be successful as a nurse. If they're providing you feedback it's most of the time, and hopefully in every case it's from a place of love and of concern where they want you to be successful.

One thing that all nurses want on their floors are nurses that are able to take care of themselves, able to take care of patients, and able to make the workload lighter on any given day. Understand that anytime you're getting feedback it's for that reason. The best thing you can do when you get feedback is just to listen, to take note of it, and to ask questions, ask, "Okay, well, how can I improve upon that?" Or, "What can I do to get better with that?" If your preceptor is telling you, "You know, you're doing a really good job but I noticed you're taking a long time to chart."

The best thing you can do is to not get offended, realize you're new, it's okay, it's okay that you're learning, that there's areas that you need to improve upon, every nurse has things they can improve upon regardless of how long they've been working. When feedback is given, take a minute and say, "Okay, well, what can I do to chart better? Have you noticed any areas that I maybe need to improve upon?" Really dig in and ask the questions of what you can do better rather than getting offended, or getting your feelings hurt, just ask what you can do better.

Don't get prideful just accept that feedback as someone trying to help you, and realize that you can grow if you take it as an opportunity to learn and to grow.

Every Employee of the Hospital Has the Same Goal

Nursing encompasses an art, a humanistic orientation, a feeling for the value of the individual, and an intuitive sense of ethics, and of the appropriateness of action taken.

— Myrtle Aydelotte, PhD, RN, FAAN

For some reason we nurses like to think that our way of doing things is the right way and the only way.

I get it . . . we take great pride in our work and accept a huge amount of responsibility for our patients and their care. This can be a very good thing. It drives us to work hard and to provide the highest level of care to our patients.

Unfortunately, this can also be a negative trait when we think that our way of doing things is the only right way.

I have found, in general, that it is best to assume that every employee at the hospital has the same goal . . . to help our patients. When you start to look for errors, scrutinize every little detail, or assume that no one is working harder than you, you are on a long road that only ends poorly.

To save yourself the stress and frustration just assume that everyone you work with has the same drive, dedication, and desire to take care of the patients as you . . . their method for carrying out that work just might be a tad different.

Where is Your Locus of Control

Whether a person is a male or female, a nurse is a nurse.

– Gary Veale, RN

Are you where you are in life as a result of choices you have made or has it been a result of luck, fate, and external forces?

This concept is referred to as "locus of control", a psychological term made popular by Julian Rotter which basically states that as humans we fall into one of two camps;

"those with an external locus of control, who believe that what happens to them is the result of chance, fate, luck and forces outside their control; and those with an internal locus of control, who believe that their life's lot is a result of their own choices and behavior"
http://www.forbes.com/sites/sebastianbailey/2014/09/17/how-changing-your-mind-can-make-you-feel-happier-earn-more-and-live-for-longer/

Being a successful nurse has a lot to do with an internal locus of control. So much can go wrong, from the moment you leave your home and drive to work until the moment you lay your head down after a long shift.

You might get a lousy assignment, you might have a patient crash, your techs and co-workers may not help you during your shift, and one of nearly a million things can go wrong during a shift. The way that you respond to these inevitable challenges will shape who you become as a nurse.

Developing an internal locus of control helps you to take responsibility for your actions and the result of those actions. On the other hand focusing on the problems, the rules, the manager that you might not get along with and blaming those external circumstances for your failures does not provide a positive solution and just gives you an excuse for your failures.

Do all that you can to develop an internal locus of control and you will go far with your career.

Keep Your Pockets Full

Nurses have come a long way in a few short decades. In the past our attention focused on physical, mental and emotional healing. Now we talk of healing your life, healing the environment and healing the planet.

-Lynn Keegan

One of the most exciting things about being a nurse is that you NEVER know what is going to happen next. That unpredictability is one of the reasons I left the mundane business world for nursing in the first place.

I will always remember a patient I received one night not too long ago. The off going nurse had stated that the patient was completely stable and oriented. Less than an hour later her pressures dropped to 70s/30s and continued to drop despite adding four vasopressors. She went from being oriented to completely incoherent, families and physicians were notified. Six nurses and two doctors spent the entire night at the patients bedside laboriously striving to determine what had happened to the patient. Intubation became inevitable and on intubation it became clear that the patient had gone into severe DIC. She continued to decline and passed away shortly after.

You never know what is going to happen.

A common phrase in nursing is "full pockets". This simply means keeping your supplies stocked, alarms set, and patient safe at all times.

Never assume you are in the clear regardless of how your patient "looks" at the moment. Fill your pocket with syringes, flushes, needles, whatever you can imagine you might need if things were to go wrong.

Not only will this save you time throughout your shift but it helps you in those critical moments if things do go wrong.

On first entering the patients room check to see that you have the supplies you need and make a mental note of anything you need to grab to have "full pockets"

Some Patients Will Never Leave You

I may be compelled to face danger, but never fear it, and while our soldiers can stand and fight, I can stand and feed and nurse them.

-Clara Barton

A lot of time is spent in nursing school brainwashing you that you should never form an emotional bond with your patients.

If you work on a busy ICU you might take care of as many as 300 patients in a single year. On a busy med-surg floor that number might be as high as 750 patients in a single year.

Once you get your feet under you and you become familiar with the diseases that you treat on your floor, patients, families, and shifts will begin to all meld into one big memory.

However, there will be some patients that you will never forget. Some patients, their stories, and their struggles will affect you so deeply that they will never leave your memory. That's okay, it doesn't make you weak. I believe that the patients that affect you this deeply are one of the blessings of being a nurse. Those patients are the ones that help you to appreciate how blessed and fortunate you are and for me, they help me to keep my feet on the ground and hug my kids a bit tighter when I return home from work.

Shortly into my career I had begun to develop pretty thick skin. Very little could happen that would shack me and most patients were forgotten the moment I clocked out at the end of my shift.

All this changed.

I walked in to a patient who was exactly my age by just a couple days, he had a baby daughter the exact same age as my little girl, he and his wife had only been married a couple of years.

This young man was suffering from encephalopathy of unknown origin and was beginning to develop a tremendous amount of cerebral edema to the point that he was completely unresponsive and was continuing to deteriorate. Neurologists, neurosurgeons, hospitalists, infectious disease, and nearly every other specialist had been brought on to the case in attempt to locate a reason for this young man's condition. No origin was discovered despite the onslaught of testing.

Over the next three days I got to know the family very closely through very intimate conversation. The patient's condition progressed very rapidly and during my last night with them the swelling progressed to the point of causing herniation and brain death.

I work on a Neuro ICU where trauma and brain death are very common but this patient and his family truly changed my life. After that shift as I left the hospital I had a completely new outlook on life. I drove over to my parents house because I couldn't wait to simply tell them I love them. I drove home and hugged my kids. A week has not passed since this experience that I have not reflected back and taken a moment to simply appreciate my life.

Some patients will stick with you forever. That's okay.

Start Your Shift With Safety Checks

Nurses are a unique kind. They have this insatiable need to care for others, which is both their biggest strength and fatal flaw.

–Dr. Jean Watson

Around 2am a few months ago I was up to receive a transfer from an outside hospital. The patient had suffered a very significant hemorrhagic stroke, meaning that she had bleeding inside her brain.

The patient was being flown in by helicopter as she was in very critical condition.

Moments later I heard the helicopter landing on the roof of the hospital. This is the moment that you know you had better be ready for your patient. Within about five minutes the elevator doors came swinging open and the flight nurses came running out of the elevator . . . tip: any time the flight nurses are running, something is WRONG!

They run full speed off the elevator and went barreling down the hall yelling "We need suction!".

The patient had aspirated and clearing her airway was vital to her survival.

Safety checks include verifying that you have the most essential equipment in your room to keep the patient safe. Here are the things that I include in my safety checks:

- 2 suction canisters with Yankauer. 1 hooked up and ready to go and another sill in package.
- The bed is locked and in the position.
- Bed alarm is on if deemed necessary.

- Alarms are set within appropriate limits for the patient.
- O2 is available.
- Lines are labeled and dated.
- Ambu bag in room.

This is obviously not a complete list of everything that needs to be done to keep a patient safe but completing this brief safety check will provide the MINIMUM standard for placing your patient in a safe environment.

I am glad that my room was ready and we were able to clear this woman's airway. The minutes required to run and grab a suction canister and set it up may have made the difference in her survival in that moment.

Push-Pause Central Lines

Our job as Nurses is to cushion the sorrow and celebrate the joy, every day, while we are 'just doing our jobs.'

-Christine Belle

Caring for central lines is different in many ways than the care of a peripheral IV.

Without covering all the needed care of a central line (you should refer to your hospitals policies and procedures for this) I simply want to be sure that you are using the most appropriate method for flushing central lines.

I am only a bit frustrated when new nurses come into the ICU and vigorously flush central lines in a hard continuous flush. When I ask if they have ever heard of "push-pause" or "pulsating flush" method for central lines, the answer I always get is, "In school we were taught that you should flush in one fast continuous flush" . . . in short . . . that is wrong.

The accepted technique for flushing central lines (including PICC lines) is a pulsating rhythm. You can refer to the recommendation from the CDC here (http://www.cdc.gov/HAI/settings/outpatient/basic-infection-control-prevention-plan-2011/central-venous-catheters.html), followed by positive pressure clamping. Again, verify this with your hospitals polices (not another nurse).

Why is the pulsating method preferred:

This method has been found to help reduce the buildup of biofilm (blood and medications) on the interior lumen of the catheter and to prevent the development of thrombus (http://www.gosh.nhs.uk/health-professionals/clinical-guidelines/central-venous-access-devices-cvads-flush-volumes/).

Positive pressure should be used when clamping the central line after a flush. This is done by simply holding pressure on your flush syringe while clamping the line at the same time. Once clamped the syringe can be removed. This aids in the reduction of blood reflux into the catheter.

Give Report by Body System

To make a difference in someone's life, you don't have to be brilliant, rich, beautiful or perfect. You just have to care.

-Mandy Hale

Nurses are trained to complete head to toe assessments. I remember how nerve racking it was in nursing school when we had to do our assessment check-offs. I might have peed my pants a little bit I was so nervous.

The head to toe assessment is vital to your job as a nurse. With time and experience you will learn to complete the assessment more effectively and quicker. It is always fun to watch an experienced nurse quickly complete their assessment while talking to the patient and without the patient even noticing.

When you give report you should do so in a head to toe fashion as well. It isn't necessary to make your report a narrative about everything that happened throughout your shift. What matters is telling the oncoming nurse exactly how the patient is NOW in a concise head to toe manner.

I have created a tool to help you organize your thoughts which you can download at NRSNG.com/54

My suggestion to you is to fill this sheet out a couple hours prior to giving your report. This will give you time to think through the most concise and clear method for giving the report.

Shift change report is hard . . . to do right. This tool will help you immensely and in no time you will be giving report like a pro.

What if it Was Your Mom

You don't build a house without its foundation. You don't build a hospital without its Nurses.

–Anonymous

You patient has pooped for the fifth time in four hours and they keep pulling out their IVs as quickly as you can put them in and they just don't feel like wearing their patient gown tonight.

This is the reality of our job.

It can be frustrating and some patients will test your patience beyond humanly possible.

In these times the best thing you can do is step out of the room, take a deep breath and think to yourself. . . what if this was my mom?

How would you treat your own mom? How would/will you want to be treated when you are the patient?

We will all age one day. We will all get sick. There is no guarantee that you or your loved one won't be the patient with severe dementia one day.

How would you expect the nurses to treat your mom if it was her in that bed?

A little empathy can go a long way.

When all else fails and my patience is exhausted . . . I start counting the hours until the end of my shift.

ABCs

Nurses quietly go about their work in a noble profession, uncelebrated soldiers toiling through the days and nights in service to the sick, the injured and the dying.

-Steve Lopez

You can simplify your job by adhering to your ABCs (airway, breathing, circulation). By organizing and prioritizing your care to address these three things in that order many decisions become much easier to make.

If you have a patient that wants water and another one who is desatting the decision is clear. Fix the airway.

If you have a stroke patient come in that is made NPO but they haven't eaten in 12 hours and keep begging you for a sandwich, stick to your ABCs. You priority as a nurse is to protect their airway.

Once the ABCs have been addressed you can move on to Maslow's hierarchy of needs. Yes, something you learned in nursing school will actually help you in your job!

For the most part as nurses our focus will remain in the physiological (ABCs) and safety realm of Maslow's.

Without sounding like I am oversimplifying nursing I will say that your ability to care for your patients and prioritize your care becomes increasingly simple if you stick with these two frameworks for decision making and prioritization.

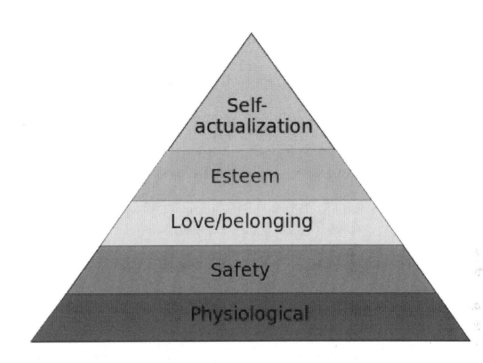

By FireflySixtySeven [CC BY-SA 4.0 (http://creativecommons.org/licenses/by-sa/4.0)], via Wikimedia Commons

Don't Judge Other Nurses

America's nurses are the beating heart of our medical system.

— President Barack Obama

When you arrive for your shift you are picking up where another nurse has been working for the past 12 hours. In this setting it can be very easy to look at everything the other nurse has done and judge their method for doing things.

Save yourself the stress and just move forward and worry about the task at hand . . . taking care of the patient.

If the room is dirty, the cables are placed a different way than you would put them, the IV poll in on the opposite side of the bed, just let it go. There is no point in judging and stressing yourself over the way that other nurses do their job.

If true concerns arise about a nurse being able to perform their job appropriately there are channels for bringing those things up but if you just want to be upset about petty things . . . let it go and move on with your job.

Carry 2 Pens and a Marker

The nurse who can smile when things go wrong is probably going off duty.

You will find that pens vanish in hospitals faster than you can imagine. I go through pens at an alarming rate. I have found that it is best to keep two pens in my front pocket at all times mostly because I know I will lose at least one throughout the shift.

Ball point pens work best because they will not smear.

It is also very helpful to keep a Sharpie marker in your pocket. These come in handy for writing on dressings, IV bags, and IV sites when needed. You may not use your Sharpie every shift but having it handy when you absolutely need it will save you a lot of stress and mislabeling.

Study for and Take Certification Tests in Your Field

Diagnosis is not the end, but the beginning of practice.

— Martin H. Fischer

Most nursing specialties have advanced certifications that you can study for and obtain.

One of the best things you can do for your career is to become a member of a nursing association or organization that administers tests in your specialty area. Being a member of these organizations will keep you up to date on new advances in your field, help you obtain CEUs, and look great on your resume.

Studying for advanced certification is one of the best ways to keep your knowledge growing. What we learn in nursing school is so general and surface that it plays little role in our ability to provide specialized care. Advanced certification is highly focused on your field and requires a depth of knowledge far beyond the NCLEX.

Passing the certification test is far less important than simply studying for it. Passing is a bonus but dedicated study will help you to obtain more focused knowledge about your patients conditions and expose you to the right literature and study guides to increase your knowledge.

When I began studying for and passed the CCRN I can honestly say that my knowledge and confidence in caring for my patients increased 100 fold.

Most hospitals will reimburse you for testing costs and some will even provide raises or bonuses for passing exams.

Ask Questions - Don't Pretend to Know

Have a heart that never hardens, a temper that never tires, a touch that never hurts.

— Charles Dickens

No one expects you to know everything as a new nurse. In fact, no one expects anyone to know everything. The great thing about nursing is that we are all always teaching each other something new.

If you aren't sure about something . . . ask! If a preceptor asks you a question and you don't know the answer . . . don't make something up!

Nothing is scarier than a new nurse who doesn't ask questions.

Asking questions doesn't mean you are an idiot, that you're unteachable, or that you will be fired. It simply means that you haven't been exposed to something, that you need a refresher, or that you need to review something.

This is the only way that more experienced nurses can know what it going on inside your mind. We have all been there and we know how much we have grown as nurses and how little we knew starting out so when a new nurses isn't asking anything we have no way of knowing what is really going on in your head and if you are thinking in the right direction.

I really can't stress this one enough . . . ASK QUESTIONS!

The most common reason I see people dismissed from our internship is simply that they are not vocal and don't ask questions.

Did you enjoy the nursing quotes in this book?

Download a PDF with all 50 Motivational Nursing Quotes HERE
(NRSNG.com/Quotes)

Your Free Gift!

As a way of saying thanks for your purchase, I'm offering a free PDF download:

"63 Must Know NCLEX® Labs"

With these charts you will be able to take the 63 most important labs with you anywhere you go!

You can download the 4 page PDF document by clicking here, or going to NRSNG.com/labs

About the Authors

Jon Haws RN CCRN: I am a registered nurse and CCRN on a Neurovascular Intensive Care Unit at a Level I Trauma Hospital. I attended college at Brigham Young University and later received my Nursing degree from Methodist College in Peoria, IL. I also hold a Business Management degree from Touro University.

Professionally, I precept nursing students and new graduate Registered Nurses and work as a charge nurse . . . and love it!

Sandra Haws MS RD CNSC: is a dietitian with one of the largest health care systems in the United States. She works with intensive care patients. She obtained her undergraduate degree from Brigham Young University and her graduate degree from Texas Woman's University. She holds advanced certifications in nutrition support management.

Visit NursingStudentBooks.com to view more books.